Critical Acclaim for J[...]
'JIM'S WEIGHT TR[...]
SUPERSET [...]

"Seeing is believing and Atkinson shows you step-by-step how to set your program up and stick with it."

– Cathy Wilson

"This is the kind of program that is finally accessible to all those who care about health and fitness."

– Grady Harp

"Jim's books take us into the world of getting fit and help to unravel the nature of each of the exercises described, based on the level or type of fitness that you are trying to achieve.
With accompanying gentle reminders to push your limits and record your progress, this book will serve as a great motivator!"

– Ryshia Kennie

" Those looking to ramp up their training have come to the right place. Atkinson makes increased fitness simple and approachable with his varied workout routines and *Supersets* training method that will increase the intensity of your workouts and improve results. Atkinson's book also gives detailed advice and images to illustrate each exercise, making the reading experience interactive and adding extra value to the instruction. I learned a lot reading this guide, and look forward to implementing Atkinson's methods into my own routine."

– B Nelson

Jim's
WEIGHT
TRAINING
GUIDE
SUPERSET STYLE

A Resistance Training Method
for Weight Loss, Muscle Growth,
Endurance *and* Strength Training

Jim's **WEIGHT TRAINING GUIDE**
SUPERSET STYLE

A Resistance Training Method
for Weight Loss, Muscle Growth,
Endurance *and* Strength Training

JAMES ATKINSON

SWAPFAT4FIT.COM
PAPERBACK EDITION

PUBLISHED BY:
JBA Publishing
http://www.swapfat4fit.com
jim@swapfat4fit.com

Book Proofing, Design & Layout by King Samuel Benson
ksb@kingsamuelbenson.com

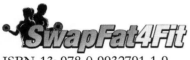

ISBN-13: 978-0-9932791-1-9

First published in 2015 / First printed in 2015
Printed in United Kingdom

TABLE OF CONTENTS

PREFACE

Hi, I'm Jim, a qualified fitness coach who is very passionate about helping people to reach their fitness potential.

During my time in the "fitness arena" I've been a long distance runner, competing bodybuilder and served a number of years in the British army in an airborne unit (9 para sqn R.E)

You will find out a lot more about me by visiting my website:

SwapFat4Fit.com

I'd like to thank you for your purchase and I know that you will get some great fitness results if you take on-board and act on the information that you read.

This book will give you many of the tools that you need to hit your fitness potential. This statement stands for all of my fitness books.

I'll let you get stuck into the book now but I would just like to let you know that if you have any questions or comments, I would be more than happy to help you as these subjects are a passion of mine and have been for many years.

If this is the first you have heard of me, great! I look forward to our training!

Although this book can be used as a stand-alone source of training guidance, the theories can also be easily incorporated into my home workout series or my other resistance training programs.

- If you are a total beginner I would advise that you start with the first book as it is a progressive fitness and fat loss workout routine specifically designed for the absolute beginner. The first book is called:
  "HOME WORKOUT FOR BEGINNERS"
- If you would rather just get stuck into this method of training, that's no problem at all. As you will see, there are many ways to use superset workouts including using them as

quick alternatives to your regular routine.

- Please be aware that some of the exercises in this book are slightly more advanced and require some form of "base training" before they can be performed correctly.
- If you have already read and completed the first six weeks home workout for beginners book, congratulations on finishing your first stage! This is a big achievement and you will no doubt be seeing the rewards from your hard work.
- If you are more advanced and are using my book:
  ## "JIM'S WEIGHT TRAINING & BODYBUILDING WORKOUT PLAN"

You will find that this guide is a good supplement to your training. If you wish to go "off-piste" and change things up a bit, you can incorporate the superset theory here to this bodybuilding guide and make it a more personal routine. If you stick to the general principals of these training theories, you can get similar results by utilising the huge range of exercise choices that are available these days.

GRAB YOUR BONUS

If you would like to be notified of any future promotions, new releases or special offers that I have on health, fitness, diet and lifestyle, please sign up to my mailing list.

I promote every e-book on its release at $0.99 or even free of charge and I would like to offer these opportunities to my loyal readers.

Why would I do this? First off, it is a "thank you" from me for choosing to buy my book over all of the competition.

And secondly, because I am an independently published author and I hold all the cards when it comes to promotion as well as writing the actual book; so the more hands that I can put my book into, the better—and why shouldn't my existing customers be amongst this special group of people?

Don't worry; I hate spam emails, too, and I get my fair share. Because of this, I rarely send out emails; but when I do, it will be something worth your while.

Please follow the link below to grab your 7 Free Healthy and Tasty Recipes that I have created myself. This free gift will help you out even more with your health and fitness plans, and it also serves as a big thank you from me for your support.

Simply enter the below website address in your browser, click "GO" or tap ENTER, and let me know where to send them!

http://swapfat4fit.com/reader-bonus/

CHAPTER 1

HOW TO GET THE MOST OUT OF THIS BOOK

Because there are many different ways to train with resistance exercise and there are many different goals that can be aspired to, i.e. bodybuilding, endurance, fat loss, etc., the full contents of this book may not be relevant to everyone.

If you are looking for ideas to use superset training to attain results in different areas of fitness, the full content will be useful; but if you are looking for ideas on using superset training for the area of fitness that you are currently involved with, you will probably be able to skip a few chunks of content and revisit it again if you change your fitness goals at a later date.

The book has been split into four sections:

SECTION 1:

Covers some of the fundamentals in resistance training. These fundamentals are not only relevant to superset training but they will serve as a solid foundation on which to build any resistance workout routine. Some of this information may also be a nice memory refresher to the basic principles behind weight training for the veteran.

SECTION 2:

Covers a selection of example superset workout routines that can be followed directly from the book or modified to suit your personal needs / goals. Some of these example routines may not be relevant to everyone. If you are not interested in some of the training effects outlined, skipping past this information is not a big deal, although it might be useful to see how supersets are employed in different training situations. This might give you some ideas when it comes to designing your own bespoke training plan.

SECTION 3:

Gives you all of the information that you need to start planning your own superset training plan. If you wish to follow one of the workout plans that were covered in the previous section, feel free to skip this section. I would advise, however, that you do take a look as there may be something in here that will encourage you to modify your workout plan to make it a bit more bespoke. Even a few little tweaks here and there can make a big difference in the long run.

SECTION 4:

This is the section with the exercise descriptions. All of the exercises that are mentioned in the example workout routines are illustrated here. Each exercise description has at least two clear studio quality photographs showing the various stages of the exercise, along with a written account of how to perform the movement safely and correctly. Please have a look at these even if you normally use these exercises on a regular basis already. We are all guilty of falling into bad habits when it comes to exercise form and I believe that performing any resistance exercise correctly is one of the top priorities of any workout routine.

Section
1

CHAPTER 2

HEALTH CHECK

Before you embark on any change of diet or fitness programme, please consult your Doctor if you are unsure of the health implications these changes may have.

- Do not exercise if you are unwell.
- Stop if you feel pain, and if the pain does not subside, then see your Doctor.
- Do not exercise if you have taken alcohol or had a large meal in the last few hours.
- If you are taking medication, please check with you Doctor to make sure that it is okay for you to make these changes.
- If in any doubt at all, please check with your Doctor first. It may be helpful to ask for a blood pressure, cholesterol and weight check. You can then have these read again in a few months after exercise or change of diet so you can monitor the benefit.
- It is also a good idea to take this workout routine with you and go through it with your doctor or physician. These guys will be able to tell you if there are any aspects that need changing based on your individual requirements.

CHAPTER 3

INTRODUCTION
WHAT ARE SUPERSETS?

Shortly after the creation of fire but before man invented the wheel, there was a clever little training method developed that was called "Supersets".

As you can see from this brief but accurate account of the origin of supersets, this manner of fitness training has been around for a long time. Like everything else in life, when something has been around for a while, it tends to develop and evolve -- and superset training is no exception to this rule.

I have seen superset exercises used in all types of training by all types of trainers and gym rats alike. But due to the lack of structure in this training, I have noticed that, on many occasions, the result or training effect would be far from optimal.

In other words: Why bother training in a certain way if it's not really going to make a difference?

First things first; what is superset training? In the simplest terms, superset training is:

"A sequence of two exercises performed directly after each other with no rest."

It is fairly safe to say that a huge percentage of the population that have trained or looked at examples of different fitness routines will be familiar with the concept of superset training.

But I know from experience that a huge proportion of these guys will not know how to utilize the superset method of training to its full potential. It seems that the usual approach to using superset training is to randomly throw it in on certain muscle groups and training days.

Yes, training in this way will not do you any harm and will almost certainly enhance your workout, but you can achieve so much more with a bit of understanding, planning and structure.

If you are interested in getting the most out of your training in general, you will no doubt find some useful information in this book that will help you get the most out of your workouts and actually achieve the training effect that you are personally looking for.

It is my intention to help you understand how to use this method of training to its full potential by means of a logical outlook. With this knowledge, you will:

- Be able to identify the workload that best suits your training goal.
- Effectively add supersets to your existing workouts.
- Use the method "full time".
- Plan to use supersets to target your weaknesses.
- Be in a position to devise your own workout routine.

So before you pick up your weights, resistance bands or start banging out body weight exercises, it is important that you understand a few basic principles that will help you fathom out how you can effectively use supersets to hit your personal fitness goals.
I would like to also point out that the theories and exercise routines that are outlined in this book are my own creation based on my education in the health and fitness field and on my personal experience. The exercise routines are generic and designed with idealism in mind. But with the accompanying information, any resistance trainer can adapt the routines to suit their specific needs.

CHAPTER 4

THE TRAINING EFFECT

You can use superset training to great effect in many different ways. But like all training methods out there, it pays to be structured and logical in your approach.

The term "training effect" does exactly what it says on the tin. But I will explain anyway:

"The training effect is the effect on your physical condition that you wish to achieve through your fitness routine and workout plans."

This means that if you want to train for fat loss, you would devise and follow a workout plan specifically optimized for fat loss. And if you wanted to gain lots of muscle mass, you would devise and follow a plan specifically designed for this purpose.

To put it a bit more simply, an extreme example would be: if you wanted to be a competition bodybuilder, you would hit the gym and lift weights; you would not go out and start long distance running.

It is with this mindset that you should approach superset training. If you want to achieve your target training results, it is helpful to know that there is a bit more to superset training than simply performing two exercises with minimal rest between sets.

CHAPTER 5

WHY USE SUPERSETS IN YOUR TRAINING?

There are many reasons that you might want to use supersets in your training routine.

Whether you want to go "full-time" with superset training, you want to hit a quicker workout once in a while or you want to incorporate superset training into your workout program once per week, by adding this training concept to your arsenal of fitness knowledge, you will find that you can increase variation and value to your training in general.

TIME SAVING

One of the most common and practical reasons for using supersets is the time-saving potential that this method of training can have. In theory and indeed practice, a trainer can nearly cut the time it takes to do a standard workout in half whilst keeping the training intensity high.

BREAK THINGS UP A BIT

Self-motivation is one of the most important factors when it comes to achieving great fitness results and it is all too common for new trainers in particular to fall victim to lack of motivation. This leads to lack of consistency, which, in turn, leads to fitness results slowing down or even taking backward steps.

Superset training sessions can come in handy at this point. If you are particularly tired or unmotivated, and are in the "should-I-give-today's-training-session-a-miss" zone at any point (let's face it; this is a common place to be and everyone will be here at one point or another), you can opt for a short, sharp training session that will not dilute the training effect that you are after, provided that you stick to your workload. (More on that later.)

Superset training can also be a refreshing change to the "everyday grind" of a regular resistance training routine. Believe it or not, a superset training session can really help to break things up a bit and boost motivation.

GET MORE DONE IN YOUR NORMAL WORKOUT TIME

If you train using the superset method for one hour, you will effectively have done the same exercise workload as nearly two hours of standard training.

This is great for high intensity training and can also be a good "comeback" if you have missed a training session earlier in the week and you would like to get this missed session in, to chalk it up as "done" on your training chart.

Yes! I believe that if you are serious about getting fitness results, you should plan ahead and make yourself a tick chart to mark off your training sessions as you complete them. This is great for accountability as well as motivation.

HIGHER INTENSITY

Because of the nature of this method of training, the workout intensity of a superset compared to a standard resistance set is much higher. This is great news for most trainers who are looking to challenge their body that little bit more.

With a regular injection of higher intensity training added to a workout routine, you can expect to get your desired fitness results in a shorter time, provided that you stick to the correct workload in relation to your specific fitness goals.

CHAPTER 6

WORKLOAD

I have used the term "workload" several times so far already in this book and stressed how important this is when it comes to achieving your desired "training effect".

I feel that the most universal way to explain the importance of using the correct workload for any given individual is that it can relate to something as simple as a shopping trip.

Stick with me here – it will all become clear!

Let's say that I wanted to go grocery shopping and I needed to get a bunch of healthy food for my new healthy lifestyle. There are a few ways that I could go about this:

A. I could head to the shops and just pick out what I thought was good-looking healthy food.

B. I could plan my diet for the week, write a list of everything that I needed and buy everything that was on the list.

If I went with option "A", I would save a fair bit of time because I didn't need to research and plan, but this is the only positive point to be gained by going down this road. I would no doubt make the wrong choices, be drawn to impulse purchases, likely forget any plan that I may have had, and I would end up with things that I didn't really want, and the whole week of "healthy living" would be ruined or, at best, sub-standard.

Option "B", however, is the way to go. By researching and planning what needs to be done in order to hit a fitness goal (or any goal for that matter), I will have a solid base and a good start. Once my planning is done, I would create a list of everything that I need from my shopping trip. Once I hit the store, I would be able to work through my list and check off exactly what I needed. I will also have an easier time with less distraction. Another plus here is that I would only really need to do the research and planning once. In the future, I would only have to tweak my plan slightly. But the biggest plus for option "B" is that I would actually be working efficiently towards a goal that I wanted to achieve.

This little shopping anecdote is a great metaphor to use in the fitness training process that many people will fall foul of.

Yes, it will all start with good intentions, but without a proper plan, there will be too many distractions and any hopes of training success will likely be doomed from the beginning.

This is why I have added the workload section to this book.

When it comes to resistance training, there are many different approaches, training methods and styles, and it is very easy to get knocked off course when looking at internet forums or even chatting to others in the gym. Again, this is a good reason to learn the workloads that you should be working with when it comes to achieving your personal fitness aspirations.

If you would like to hit your personal fitness goals in the most efficient way, you need to understand the workloads that you train with. For the purpose of this book, workloads will be primarily based on the concept of sets, reps and resistance level.

For example: If you want to become a muscle-bound hulk, you would not do 25-50 reps of 5 sets on isolation exercises only.

And on the other end of the scale: If you wanted to be an endurance athlete and compete in ironman challenges, you would not hit the heavy compound exercises like squats and deadlifts for sets of 10.

As this book is mainly aimed at resistance exercise routines, we will keep to a workload that I understand to be optimal for different fitness goals. I also believe that this workload knowledge is a fundamental part of hitting personal fitness development aspirations in the most efficient way possible.

If this book is your first introduction to the world of resistance training, here are some definitions to make this section a bit clearer:

DEFINITIONS EXPLAINED

Sets:
The amount of times that you will perform a set number of repetitions (reps) of a given exercise.

Reps:
The number of repetitions (reps) of the same exercise movement in any given set.

Isolation exercises:
An exercise that targets a single muscle group. Isolation exercises usually only use one body joint movement per rep. A few examples of these are dumbbell raises and pec flyes.

Compound Exercises:
An exercise that targets several muscle groups. Compound exercises usually use more than one body joint movement per rep. A few examples of these exercises are any press movements such as shoulder press, chest press and also big exercises like squats.

Resistance level:
The resistance of the exercise being performed. This can be measured in weight of dumbbells, barbells, bodyweight or resistance bands. Resistance can be measured as "% of max weight".

To gauge your personal "% max" on an exercise, you should do a simple test. This type of testing is mainly used for compound movements, but it can also be used for isolation exercises. If you do wish to test your % max on any isolation exercise, you should take extra care as heavy weights on this type of exercise can have a higher risk of injury.

The most accurate way of finding out your personal "max weight" is:

- Warm your body up fully. The best way to do this is by doing a 10 – 15 minutes session on a cross trainer. A cross trainer will get your entire body ready for a workout. Equipment like stationary bikes will not do such a great job but are still viable.

- Once you are warm, go to your first exercise and perform a warm up set of about 20 - 30 reps with a very light resistance level. This is to ensure that the muscle that you are working is completely warm.
- Staying with this exercise choice, you should increase the weight and perform 1 rep using very strict form. Try to be ambitious with your weight choice.
- Keep adding weight and performing a set of 1 rep between weight additions until you hit a set where you can no longer lift with strict form. The last set that you did with strict form signifies the weight of your "% max" for that exercise.
- Repeat this process for every exercise in your routine and make a note of each exercise and % max weight. Bear in mind that the more consistent your training is, the stronger you will become so you may want to repeat this process every 4 – 6 weeks to see if your % max has increased.
- It is important that you keep your lifting form as strict as possible when testing for your % max resistance on every exercise.

Testing your % max on exercise choices may seem like a bit of a geeky thing to do but this information is valuable and it is a good measure when it comes to working with the correct weight for optimum results. For the purpose of this book we will use "% max" as part of the workload.

The longer that you are in the resistance game, and the more that you develop, the more you will learn about your strengths and weaknesses.

Workload:
The workload is a general term for the amount of sets, reps and resistance per exercise. For example, the workload of a strength training squat session would be:

"3 sets of 10 reps. Resistance should be heavy enough so failure is reached at 10 reps and not before."

Training days:
You should tailor your training days according to your desired training effect when it comes to resistance exercise. Believe it or not, some forms of training only need to be done a few days per week whereas others will have a higher frequency.

For example: If you are into strength training, you can train on a full body routine only 3 times per week with a fairly weighty workload. But if you are looking to burn fat, you will benefit from training everyday with a less intense workload.

Here is a guide to help you determine your training days based on the training effect that you require:

Please note that this is a general approach and most certainly not the definitive guide. There are many ways that you can adapt your training days by using split routines, full body, blitzing or any other method.

GENERAL FITNESS:
3 – 7 full body resistance and cardio training sessions per week.

STRENGTH:
3 full body training sessions per week.

BODYBUILDING:
4 – 6 split training sessions per week.

ENDURANCE AND STAMINA:
5 – 7 split or full body training sessions per week.

FAT BURNING:
5 – 7 full body resistance and cardio training sessions per week.

CHAPTER 7

WHICH WORKLOAD IS FOR YOU?

By understanding the workload of the training effect that you are looking for, you will be in a better position to devise your own effective training routine using supersets or otherwise.

Here is a description of the training workloads for different training effects:

GENERAL FITNESS

General fitness covers fat loss, muscle tone and basic muscular function. If you are new to fitness and fat loss, this is where you should start.

You should always start with a general fitness workout routine even if your ambitions are set to become an elite fitness trainer such as an ultra-marathon runner or, at the other end of the scale, a competing bodybuilder. The general fitness workload is a sensible starting point for any new trainer.

GENERAL FITNESS WORKLOAD:
2-3 sets
12-15 reps
50% of max resistance
3 – 7 days per week

STRENGTH

A strength training routine is a natural progression from a general fitness training routine. In my opinion (I may be bias, as this is where it all began for me), strength training is one of the best forms of resistance exercise for almost everyone. It is a natural progression from general fitness and it also goes hand-in-hand with bodybuilding routines.

Strength training is often overlooked and undervalued. This is probably because the majority of individuals who decide to start a lifestyle of fitness do this for atheistic or general health reasons and real strength training does not seem to offer any of these benefits directly.

In reality, strength training is a great catalyst to achieving better than average results. For example: If you want to become a bodybuilder and you go right into a bodybuilding routine, you will not have the muscular strength to perform the optimal workload for a bodybuilding routine so your results will be diluted a fair bit.

On the other hand, if you decided to become a bodybuilder and your first thought was to build up your strength to be able to hit the training intensity and volume that is optimum for building quality muscle, you would have very good results and your training time would be spent most efficiently in this situation.

STRENGTH TRAINING WORKLOAD:
3 sets
10 reps
70 – 85% Max resistance
3 days per week

BODYBUILDING

Bodybuilding training is a good progression from strength training as the strength that has been developed during this time will really help to boost results in the bodybuilding game.

Unlike strength training, with bodybuilding training, the trainer must have a slightly different mindset when it comes to working out. If you want to hit a bodybuilding training routine, you should understand that the training sessions will have more volume, they will be more intense and each muscle group will be pushed with more repetition and focus.

Although it is true for all areas of fitness to state that nutrition is important if you want to achieve the desired training effect, it is never truer with bodybuilding. Correct nutrition and bodybuilding go together like peas and carrots! Or indeed chicken and rice.

One more point about bodybuilding that I will make is that bodybuilding training routines are not just for guys and gals who want to look like Arnold or The Rock. Bodybuilding routines can be used for fitness models, fat loss and can be used as a progression from general fitness. So, although bodybuilding training is generally used to bulk up, it can also be used for body sculpting to great effect.

It is extremely rewarding to see your body change and develop through any type of workout routine, but bodybuilding training can target specific areas and this is your best chance at earning your potential in aesthetic bodily perfection.

BODYBUILDING WORKLOAD:
4 - 6 sets
12 - 8 reps
70 – 75% Max resistance
4 – 6 days per week

ENDURANCE / STAMINA

Endurance and stamina training can be a progression from any of the other workout methods, but it is most natural to progress from a general fitness or fat burning routine.

The main point to note about endurance and stamina training is the diverse rep range that can be done per exercise set. There is huge scope for development in this area. For example: you can change the resistance level so you can work at a higher rep range, and it is because of this rep range that you can devise a fairly varied structure to your training routine.

Endurance training can be tough and the more mentally robust that you can make yourself, the better your development will be. It is all too easy for a trainer to say;

"I can't do any more, that's me at my limit"

But if you decide to take up the challenge of stamina and endurance training and you actually want good results. You should bring your "I can always do one more rep!" head with you. Just like Rocky!

ENDURANCE / STAMINA WORKLOAD:
3 sets
15 - 50 reps
60% Max resistance
5 – 7 days per week

FAT BURNING

I will go right ahead and say that fat burning results can come from most forms of training. But if you are looking to burn fat as your priority in terms of training effect, there is an optimum way to do this.

There are many different opinions on the best way to burn fat. This means that there are also contradictions. I have personal experience with extreme fat burning and managed to get myself down to a single figure body fat %. I have also tried a few different methods, but I will share the rules from my most successful endeavors.

If burning fat is your sole priority when it comes to training, there are a few factors that you should consider:

1. The more muscle that you have on your body, the more calories your body will burn per workout session and at rest.
2. The more exercise that you do, the more calories you will burn.
3. The less refined sugar and saturated fat that you eat, the less fat you will gain.
4. The more calories that you eat in general and do not burn off, the more fat you will retain.
5. The workout intensity should be slow and steady rather than "explosive and brutal". The main reason for this is that good fat burning results come from very regular and consistent workouts. So if your workout routine is too punishing, your body will less likely be able to sustain this regular vigor before giving in to injury.
6. In most people, the optimal fat burning heart rate is lower than that of cardio endurance training. This means that you can get good fat burning results from longer, less intense

training sessions.

As you can see from some of the points on the list, exercise is one thing but diet is another and nutrition is a whole new beast. This book is all about exercise, so this will be our focus, but please don't neglect your diet.

A great starting point with diet is making yourself aware of the amount of "bad calories" you are eating on a daily basis. Make a daily food diary of everything that you put in your mouth and look at this at the end of a week. You might be surprised.

If you are looking to train for fat burning, using circuit training is slightly different to any of the other training effects in that it is more dynamic.

Going back to the exercise side of things now; as you can see, the more muscle that we have, the more efficiently our body will burn calories. So it makes sense to use resistance exercise to stimulate our major muscle groups for an optimum fat burning workout.

We also know that the more exercise that we do, the more calories we will burn. So it makes sense to make the most of our workout sessions by keeping them flowing and continuous.

If we combine these two fat burning ideas, we come to another of my favorite workout methods called "circuit training". This is the subject of one of my other books called:

"Home Workout Circuit Training"

Just like superset training, circuit training is a Pandora's box of potential scope for ideas and training variation, and as I have covered some in-depth circuit training workout routines in my other book, I will cover a basic idea here where superset training can be used.

The first difference with a superset fat burning routine is that you can choose to work with a "timed" set rather than performing a set with a fixed number of reps. For example; instead of performing a set of 15 reps, you perform a set of 30 seconds.

Timed sets are great if you are proficient at performing the exercise choices and I would advise that this is the way to go should you choose a "superset circuit for fat burning".

If you are totally new to training in general or the exercise choices that you will be using in your workout, it is a good idea to start off with the more standard "fixed number" sets. This will help you perfect the movement and strengthen the muscles being worked. The training will also help you get the most out of your timed sets when you progress as you will not be concentrating on getting your exercise form up to scratch and your focus can be on the bigger picture.

Here are a few points to note if you decide to hit these circuits with timed sets:

- Remember the max resistance for fat burning is only 50%, so you can train with more consistency and for longer.
- You should choose a resistance level or weight that allows you to perform your workload comfortably but is still challenging to you.
- When you perform resistance exercises, you should keep the movement flowing with each full rep lasting 4 seconds (2 seconds from start to mid and 2 seconds from mid back to start).
- Find a rhythm in your breathing throughout your workout, and, on most resistance exercises, you should breathe out on the effort.

One more difference with this type of training is a thing that I like to call "active rest".

It may sound like a contradiction, but active rest is a great way to keep your body temperature up and your body actually burning fat between sets. Although you can choose to train for fat burning with a short rest in-between supersets, there is a way to use this time to your advantage and further increase the fat burning potential of your workout.

After each superset, instead of sitting down, looking in the mirror and flexing to see how amazing your results have been so far or just standing still and psyching yourself up for the next set, you can actually have a timed "rest set" of light cardio.

This is not as bad as it sounds. The cardio could be a simple step up, step down using an exercise step or even a breeze block. The light constant cardio will keep your core temperature up, keep you focused and keep you in your fat burning zone. As these "rest sets" will be timed, your workouts will also be more dynamic and flowing with less chance of distraction. All of this will make for a very efficient fat burning workout.

FAT BURNING WORKLOAD:

3 - 4 sets

12 – 25 standard reps or timed 30 seconds – 1 minute reps

50% Max resistance

5 - 7 days per week

CHAPTER 8

CORRECT FORM ALWAYS

When you perform any exercise whether it is cardio or resistance, it is important to maintain correct exercise form.

For the benefit of first-time trainers; correct exercise form means that you perform an exercise in the safest, most functional way possible. You should be targeting the muscle group that you want to develop as an outcome of that exercise whilst also maintaining good posture to avoid injury.

Correct exercise form is an extremely important part of any training routine. If the form of an exercise is consistently performed incorrectly, over time, a trainer can actually cause their body serious damage.

Training with incorrect form over a period of time can cause muscle shortening which in turn causes loss of range of motion in joint movements, tendon and ligament weakness and you can also train yourself into a bad posture.

So it is important to understand that injuries that happen in the gym are not all sudden and excruciating bolts of pain that can put an instant stop to your training. Some of the injuries will be far more insidious.

This is why you should pay attention to your exercise form from the word "go". You should also revisit and constantly check your form through the full life of your training.

I, myself, have been training in the gym for many years using the core exercises like squats, bench press, barbell shoulder press, etc. since I started and I even teach these exercise choices to others. But it is not uncommon for me to check and adjust my own form or even ask other personal trainers to check my form from time to time.

Just because I am a teacher does not make me immune to bad habits.

If you, too, have been training for a while and not paid that much attention to exercise form, I would advise that you make this a priority. It is a good idea to start with the exercises that you are already doing on a regular basis.

Be aware that if you have trained for a while and are just now starting to concentrate on strict exercise form, your workload on that exercise might drop significantly.

Please don't be put off by this reduced workload, it is important to understand that it is not your strength or anything else that has diminished. It is simply because you have a less diluted training technique and the muscle group that you are targeting is actually working harder.

As this book has example workout sessions with recommended exercise choices, I have added illustrated descriptions of each exercise that is featured. You will find these exercise descriptions at the back of the book.

- Each exercise has two illustrations (there are some exceptions). The first is the "start position" and the second is the "mid position".
- Each exercise description shows and describes how to perform a single rep of that exercise.
- Each exercise description takes you through start position to mid position and back to start position. Breathing and tempo is also explained.

As mentioned earlier, exercise form is an extremely important part of fitness training and, in my opinion, should be a priority in any trainer's fitness endeavor.

So I would advise that you revisit the description of any exercise choices that you decide to use in your training on a regular basis. It is also wise not to become overly confident in your ability to perform the exercise choices that you use on a regular basis. Bad habits can creep in easily if you stop questioning your form.

CHAPTER 9

A STRUCTURED APPROACH TO TRAINING

A huge factor in the level of success that can be earned from physical training is determined by the structure and planning of a training routine based on the desired training effect.

All too often, someone will hear or read about a certain training method that "sounds like fun" and they will go to the gym and put it into practice "here and there".

Training in this way is okay and you will still benefit from the exercise but if you take a bit of time to put a plan together, you will no doubt benefit ten times over with this structure to your workouts.

My philosophy is that; if you decide to start working out, go to the gym or even just force yourself to do your first one-off cardio session, your actions state that you want to improve on a certain aspect of your fitness. So if you are motivated enough to act at all, you may as well make your training sessions count.

Before you start any type of training routine or even training method such as supersets, I would always advise that you make the most out of it by sitting down and putting a plan together.

The time that you spend in planning will not only help you develop physically, but it will spur you on mentally. With a training plan that is designed with your personal needs in mind, you will have a big head start and your sessions will be more efficient at helping you get the training results that you are looking for.

So, what do you do first? The first thing that you should do is decide what you want to achieve as a result of your training. In a previous section, we looked at "the training effect" and the different workloads that you should follow to achieve the appropriate effect: If you want to burn fat, you should use a fat burning workload. If you want to build strength, you should use a strength training workload, etc.

Once you have decided what type of training effect you want to achieve, the next thing is to decide which days of the week you can train. It is a good idea to get a "Training calendar" set up so you can plan each training session for several future weeks and tick them off as you go. This also serves as an accountability aid.

Using your chosen workload, you should plan at least eight weeks ahead on this calendar. In my experience, eight weeks is a good timescale to measure results from most training routines. Any less and you may not have given the training effect a good enough chance to start working.

Section
2

CHAPTER 10

SUPERSETS FOR STRENGTH & MASS

If you are looking to build strength and mass, you should aim to be hitting mainly compound movements and your target should be reaching failure at about the tenth rep of each set.

It may take you a few workouts-worth of experimenting with different workloads, i.e. amount of weight you are lifting per exercise, but this is a fundamental part of making progress in the game of "Strength and Mass".

I always find that gaining strength and mass is a good starting point for most macro cycles. (A macro cycle is years' worth of training set out with a final goal in mind.)

By starting with Strength training, you will be creating a good foundation for future development in all other areas of fitness. So it's only fitting that we will look at this type of superset training first.

As well as using compound movements with this type of training, it's a good idea to also aim at opposing muscle groups per superset. For example: chest (pectorals) will be worked with back (latissimus dorsi); front of upper arms (biceps) will be worked with rear upper arms (triceps) etc.

Because of the all-over nature of this training, if you do wish to go "fulltime", I would advise that you only hit this exercise routine three times in any given week whilst spacing out your workouts with at least one day rest between each session.

So, ideally, you would only train on Mondays, Wednesdays and Fridays.

If you do feel that this is not enough, you could fill the missing days with abdominal workouts or light cardio sessions.

Below is an example of a *supersets for strength and mass* workout:

Chest / Back
Chest press / Bent over rows

Quads / Hamstring
Hack Squats / Stiff legged deadlifts

Biceps / Triceps
Barbell bicep curls / Close grip bench press

Shoulders / Calves
Shoulder press / Calve raises

Abs / Lower back *(optional but advised)*
Swissball crunches / Dorsal raises

3 sets, 10 reps

CHAPTER 11

SUPERSETS FOR STAMINA & TONING

If the main focus of your training is to develop stamina and muscle tone, you would benefit from a different approach to superset training than Strength & Mass or Fat Burning.

Although training for stamina and muscle tone will also help with fat loss, there is a way to optimize your training so it leans more towards stamina and muscle toning as a priority.

In my personal experience and training, I have learned that the basic rules in achieving stamina and muscle tone as a training effect are pretty simple, like all of the other "training effect" concepts.

The basic idea is that high reps and sets of an exercise will develop stamina. This high volume training method can be used to target single muscle groups, full body movements or indeed cardiovascular exercise choices.

As this book is aimed at mainly resistance training, we will look at how we can exploit the superset workout method to develop stamina and muscle tone through these means.

If you do set out to work on stamina and muscle tone, I feel that it is worth mentioning that muscle tone is a "by product" of the stamina.

By doing this type of training and workload, you will find that your body will become leaner and defined but if the visual aesthetics of your body is more important to you than the function, you would probably benefit more from a bodybuilding training routine.

This full body workout is a mix of isolation and compound movements and due to increased reps, resistance will need to be lighter.

Chest / Back
Pushups / Seated rows (exercise band)

Quads / Hamstring
Squats / Lunges

Biceps / Triceps
Bicep curls / Close grip pushups

Shoulders / Calves
Lateral raises / Calve raises

Abs / Lower back *(optional but advised)*
Swissball crunches / Dorsal raises

4 sets, 15 - 25 reps

CHAPTER 12

SUPERSETS FOR FAT BURNING

If your main reason for training is to burn fat, then you can really utilize a superset routine to ensure this training effect.

The first thing that you need to understand is that the fat burning potential of this type of workout is very great. If you have done any of the other methods of superset training, this particular one is slightly different so you may need a slight shift in mindset to fully grasp superset training for fat burning.

For this example, I will outline a simple routine and advise on an upgrade.

This style of training will utilize timed sets of a mixture of compound, isolation and light cardio exercises.

The idea behind this is that you keep your body moving for a set time, and, by using these movements, you will be employing several muscle groups. Training in this way is a bit more demanding on the whole body and it means that you will be burning more calories than you would if you were simply doing several sets and reps of an exercise.

Because of the workout intensity and constant movements, you should select a weight or "workload" on these resistance exercises that is challenging but not too heavy. If you find that you can't finish the routine or you can't get through the full timed set, you should look to decrease the workload used.

This is an example of a "Supersets for fat burning" workout:

30 seconds – 2 minutes per exercise with 30 seconds – 1 minute "active rest set" between supersets. You should follow the list of exercises from 1 – 10 without stopping and count each full pass as 1 set. Once that you have completed a full set, have a 2 minutes water break and then continue.

1. **Full pushups or pushups on knees / Seated rows (exercise band)**

2. Active rest (Step ups)

3. **Bodyweight Squats / Lunges**

4. Active rest (Step ups)

5. **Bicep curls / Tricep dips**

6. Active rest (Step ups)

7. **Lateral raises / Shoulder press**

8. Active rest (Step ups)

9. **Crunches / Dorsal raises**

10. Active rest (Step ups)

3 – 6 sets
30 seconds – 2 minute per exercise

FAT BURNING UPGRADE

This is a slight upgrade. I have changed the exercise choices making them a bit more challenging.

It may look like a small upgrade that is hardly worth doing but in the fat burning game, these little tweaks are what can make a world of difference.

You can determine the intensity of your workout at this point by changing the tempo of your "Rest set". Up the tempo and you up your results!

Although it is true to say, "The harder that you work, the better your results," but you must also be sensible. There is no point burning yourself out on your first rest set. Doing this would kill your workout and it will actually be detrimental to your progress.

If you do wish to try these fat burning workout methods, I would suggest that you start off with a very slow tempo on these rest sets and then step it up a notch with each future training session until you are at a steady jog. If you are feeling particularly energetic and dedicated, you may even want to throw in a few sprints.

This is what the upgrade looks like:

1. Step ups (Rest set)

2. **Pushups / Bench jumps**

3. Step ups (Rest set)

4. **Squats / Alternate squat thrusts**

5. Step ups (Rest set)

6. **Bicep curls / Alternate squat thrusts**

7. Step ups (Rest set)

8. **Bench dips / Crawling steps**

9. Step ups (Rest set)

10. **Crunches / Star jumps**

11. Step ups (Rest set)

3 – 6 sets
30 seconds – 2 minute per exercise

Section 3

CHAPTER 13

ADDING SUPERSETS TO YOUR CURRENT WORKOUT ROUTINE

It is likely that most people reading this book would like to get a taste for this method of training by trying it out in their current workout routine rather than changing the whole dynamics of their current resistance training.

This is a sensible start, and if the principals that have already been outlined are put to use, there is no reason that various superset exercises cannot be added into regular exercise routines for long term training plans.

If you are looking to go down this route and add a few supersets into the training mix, you should first look at the training effect that you want and make a logical decision on the supersets that you want to add.

For example; if I was to add a superset or two to my regular training, I would need to tailor the superset to suit a bodybuilding training effect and workload. To make this a bit more worthwhile to my specific personal needs, it would be a good idea to choose some of my weaker muscle groups to target.

With this in mind, I would probably look to hit my arms (I was at the back of the queue when arm muscles were being given out so it would pay to give these muscles a bit more attention). As my current training is focused on strength and size, I would use an "opposing muscle workout" using compound exercises with a muscle building workload:

Barbell curls / Close grip bench press
3 sets of 10 reps at 85% max resistance

As I am training these muscle groups three times per week with a view to increase my strength, I would perform this superset three times per week along with my other regular compound exercises.

This choice of superset would be ideal for my specific training needs but the great thing about this approach to training is that it is hugely diverse and supersets can be used to enhance pretty much all forms of training.

SAME MUSCLE SUPERSETS

Training the same muscle group with consecutive exercises is not only a good way to add intensity to the workout, but this will also add big training intensity to the muscle being worked.

This type of superset training, generally lends itself to bodybuilding, muscle toning and, in some cases, endurance.

You can superset any two exercises for the body part that you are targeting, but I find an isolation exercise (an exercise that uses one body joint movement to perform a single rep) followed by a compound exercise (an exercise that uses more than one body joint to perform a single rep) does wonders for this type of training.

This is actually known as a "pre exhaust set". I do go into this concept in a bit more depth with full pre exhaust exercise routines in one of my other books:

"Jim's Weight Training & Bodybuilding Workout Plan"

So I won't start to get boring by repeating myself.

It is also a good idea to target your weak body parts if you only intend to try this concept out or want to start weaning supersets into your regular routine.

So if you decide that you want to, maybe, add a bit of muscle mass, or you want to tone and shape a particular body part, supersets on the same muscle group with a pre exhaust concept thrown in would be ideal for your training needs.

Once you have decided you want to have a go at this, you should confirm your workload and identify the body part that you would like to improve. For this example, I will use shoulders (deltoids) and I will tailor this to a bodybuilding routine:

Lateral raises / Shoulder press
4 sets of 12 reps at 75% max resistance

As you can see; lateral raises is an isolation exercise for the shoulders and shoulder press is a compound exercise for the shoulders. If you are unsure how to perform any of these exercises, please check the exercise descriptions at the back of the book.

As mentioned earlier, this superset can be used to sculpt and tone as well as build muscle mass. If this was your goal, you could still use the same two exercises as part of the superset but you would need to change the workload accordingly.

OPPOSING MUSCLE SUPERSETS

This has been briefly covered, using myself as an example, but this type of superset training is probably the most versatile as it can be used to good effect with all workloads outlined in this book.

So if you are interested in strength training and would like to throw in some supersets here and there, I would suggest that you take this approach.

Training opposing muscle groups as part of this superset is a great way to get some good compound movements in. Again, these compound exercises that target more than one muscle group are perfect for strength training.

If we are using strength training as an example for opposing muscle groups, we could select a bicep / tricep, or quadriceps / hamstrings. But in this second example, I would like to point out a common compound superset using two big compound exercises.

Barbell Chest press / Bent over barbell rows
3 sets 10 reps at 85% Max resistance

If you are unsure about these exercise choices, please check the exercise descriptions at the back of the book and you will see that this superset is a good choice for opposing muscle groups and with the workload pointed out in the example, you will be on track to develop your strength training if you choose to follow this.

As mentioned in the opening paragraph of this sub section, training with these opposing muscle supersets can be great for other training effects. Looking at the chest and back superset example above, if we keep the same exercise choices and just change the workload to a fat burning workload, this superset becomes an excellent choice as an addition to a fat burning workout. These big compound movements will help you burn off more calories than isolation movements and the added sets and reps will further support this fat burning outcome.

CHAPTER 14

THE RULES

Where do you go from here?

You could use the exercise plans that I have written directly out of this book but everyone is different; some people might be training from home, others may have access to a well-equipped gym and therefore have more scope for exercise choices and variation.

Hopefully, by this point in the book, you will have a better understanding on how to use superset training to good effect.

If you would rather use the theories behind this method of training to design a full workout or just add a superset or two to your regular training, here is a summary to follow.

If you refer to this list when creating your own structured superset master plan, you will have a much better chance of achieving good fitness results.

Refer to the numbered steps in the guide below when deciding how to use supersets in your own personal fitness journey:

1. Decide what training effect you want to achieve: fat loss, muscle gain, endurance, etc.
2. Identify your workload: sets, reps, training days, etc.
3. Plan your workout days: which day(s) will you put these into action?
4. Identify which muscle group(s) you want to develop using the superset method of training (your weaker muscle groups are a good start).
5. Decide which method of superset training you will use: same muscle group, opposing muscle groups, etc.
6. Plan your routine (exercise choices).

Stick with it for at least 6 – 8 weeks for a more accurate measure of success.

CHAPTER 15

BE CREATIVE (BUT REMEMBER)

As you can see, there are many ways that you can incorporate superset training into your resistance workouts, so there is no definitive answer to this type of training. This means that you can be very creative when it comes to your personal training style and goals.

There are, however, some effective ways to make your training more efficient; meaning that if you never forget the fundamentals of resistance training, you will be helping yourself more than you probably know.

Your form: When lifting weights, using exercise bands or performing bodyweight exercises, the first thing that you should be aware of is your form. Never sacrifice form for workload; exercise form comes first at all times.

If you are unsure how to perform any of the exercises featured in this book or any of my books for that matter, you will find a detailed description of all exercises at the back or towards the end. This description describes everything that you need to know including starting position, mid position and breathing. Sometimes, these descriptions will have more than two pictures.

Workload guidelines: Don't stray too far from the workload guidelines. We are all guilty of this and the more competitive among us can get a bit too ambitious when it comes to progression. An example of this could be a trainer with his mind set on bodybuilding goals. He may add too much resistance to his exercise choice and cause a shortfall in the amount of reps he should be doing for his target bodybuilding goal. Adding too much resistance or "weight to the bar" can also increase the chance of substandard exercise form. You should always push yourself, but it is important to stay focused on your overall goal. This may be difficult at first, but the more you practice this mentality, the more natural it will become

It also goes the other way. It's very easy to sit back and believe, because you have walked into the gym or picked up your home workout kit and decided to go through the motions and not really push yourself, that this is good enough. This is a very common training mistake that those trainers who have been gym members for years and still look the same are guilty of.

I know that this makes me sound harsh, but I believe that it is a fair comment. I view the problem like this:

If you train for one hour and go through the motions by not pushing yourself and not hitting your target workload, you will have wasted your time to some extent. You are training for an hour anyway so you should make this training session count. If you are challenging yourself on a regular basis, you will boost your training results exponentially. To adopt this mentality is a no-brainer to me and it is probably the missing link in many frustrated trainers' journey to fitness success.

It is also true to say that the longer that you practice this mindset, the easier and more natural it will become.

CHAPTER 16

WHAT TO DO NOW

If you liked my ideas and theories on superset training, great! As pleased as I am that you bought this book and actually read it, I would just like to point out that the next part is down to you.

It is the "Take Action" part. If much of this information is new to you, it may require a bit of time for you sit down and draw up a good plan. Yes, this may feel like a bit of a pain and I am willing to bet a pound to a penny that many people who have read the book with the intention of trying superset training will not actually take this time.

It is my philosophy, when it comes to fitness training, that it should be taken seriously; and the more effort that you put in, the richer the rewards will be. It also stands to reason that the longer you act in this way, the more comfortable it will become and the less hassle it will be to sit down a do a bit of "fitness planning".

Please have a look through the exercise descriptions in the following section to familiarize yourself and if you have any questions, please feel free to drop me an email: Jim@swapfat4fit.com

Section
4

EXERCISE DESCRIPTIONS

BENCH PRESS

Start Position

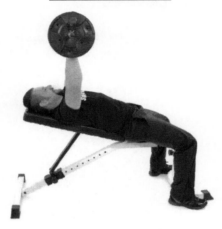

Top Of Movement

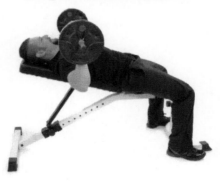

DESCRIPTION OF EXERCISE
(BENCH PRESS)

Compound exercise targeting: **Chest Muscles**

Start Position: Lay on a bench under a barbell on a rack or smiths machine so that your eyes are in line with the bar. Form a right angle with your arms. This will form your grip width. Now grip the bar.
(Note that a slight incline on the bench setting will work to target the upper chest more. I would advise that females especially should have at least a small incline on the bench.)

Movement: Lift the bar off the rack or unhook from a smiths machine and straighten your arms, ensuring you do not lock your elbows. As you inhale, lower the bar down to meet your mid chest. As the bar touches your mid chest or you reach your full range of movement, exhale and push the bar back up to the start position.
You should complete this with a 2-seconds-up-2-seconds-down tempo. This will ensure that you are getting the most out of the exercise.

BENT OVER ROWS
(SHOULDER WIDTH GRIP)

Start Position

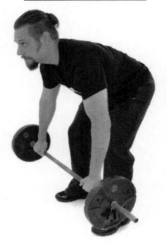

Top Of Movement

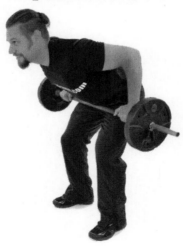

DESCRIPTION OF EXERCISE
BENT OVER ROWS (SHOULDER WIDTH GRIP)

Compound exercise targeting: **Back Muscles (Lats)**

Start position: Place your bar on the floor and stand in front of it with your feet shoulder-width apart and toes turned out slightly. Keeping your knees bent and back flat, bend over and pick up the bar. Grip the bar so your hands are in line with your outer shoulders and take a further hand space wider but no more than this.

Keeping your knees bent and back flat, stand up straight with the bar. If you need to at this point, you can adjust the width of your feet so that it is comfortable. Keeping your back flat and knees bent, lower the bar so that it hangs below your knees.

Movement: As you exhale, bring the bar up so that it touches your belly button, your elbows should go higher than your back. It is important that your back is kept flat throughout the exercise.

(I find that, when doing rows, if I concentrate on pushing my chest forward at the top of the movement, it helps to keep my back flat.)

As you exhale, lower the bar back to the starting position.

You should complete this with a 2-seconds-up-2-seconds-down tempo. This will ensure that you are getting the most out of the exercise.

HACK SQUATS

Start Position

Top Of Movement

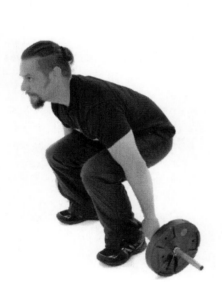

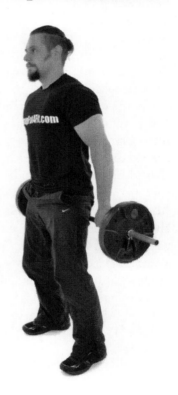

DESCRIPTION OF EXERCISE
HACK SQUATS

Compound exercise targeting: **Front Upper Leg Muscles (Quads)**

This exercise can be performed in several different ways. You can use a smiths machine, hack squat machine or even a swiss ball and barbell. But the most versatile way to do these is with a standard barbell. Performing the exercise in this way will allow you to hit this muscle group with minimum equipment and as part of a home workout.

Start position: Set up your barbell with the weight that is respective to your workload and place it on the floor. Position yourself so that the bar is behind you. Stand with your feet and knees about shoulder-width apart and perform a squat to pick up the bar. Ensure that you maintain a flat back as you slowly stand up straight. Your palms should be facing to your rear when gripping the bar. You knees should not be locked and should be slightly bent.

Movement: As you inhale, squat down until your upper legs are just above parallel to the ground (You can choose to go deeper as this will bring in your glutes, but I would not recommend squatting any lower than parallel on this movement). Once you are at your desired range of movement, exhale as you return to the starting position. Ensure that your back is straight throughout this movement.
You should complete this with a 3-seconds-up-3-seconds-down tempo. This will ensure that you are getting the most out of the exercise.

STIFF LEGGED DEAD LIFTS

Start Position

Top Of Movement

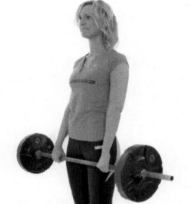

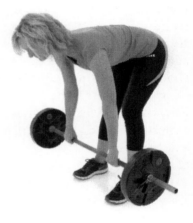

DESCRIPTION OF EXERCISE
STIFF LEGGED DEAD LIFTS

Compound exercise targeting: **Rear Upper Leg (Hamstrings)**

Start position: If you have a rack, it will help to place your bar on this to start with. Grip the bar with about a shoulder-width gap. With your back flat and knees bent, pick your bar up so it hangs just in front of your quads. Ensure that your feet are hip-width apart and are facing forward.

Movement: You do not need to keep your legs locked in a straight position. Keep your knees slightly bent, and with a flat back and arms slightly bent at the elbows, exhale as you lower the weight forward, bending at your hips. You should lower the bar to the point that you feel the stretch. This will vary from person to person. Inhale as you slowly return to the start position whilst maintaining a flat back and slightly bent knees.

You may need to stand on a step whilst doing this movement to allow the weight some ground clearance.

You should complete this with a 3-seconds-up-3-seconds-down tempo. This will ensure that you are getting the most out of the exercise.

BICEP CURLS

Start Position

Top Of Movement

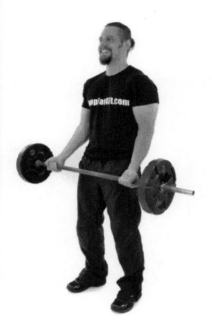

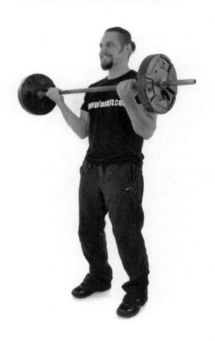

DESCRIPTION OF EXERCISE
BICEP CURLS

Compound exercise targeting: **Front Upper Arm Muscles**

Start position: When picking up your bar, ensure that your knees are bent and back is flat. When gripping the bar, your palms should be facing up and your hands should be shoulder-width apart. Stand up straight, elbows slightly bent – NOT LOCKED OUT – and you are ready to begin.

Movement: As you exhale, bring your forearms up until they are at a right angle to the floor; at this point, in one movement, push your elbows forward to bring your hands closer to the front of your shoulders. At maximum contraction, inhale as you lower the bar back to the start position.

You should complete this with a 2-seconds-up-2-seconds-down tempo. This will ensure that you are getting the most out of the exercise.

CLOSE GRIP BENCH PRESS

Start Position

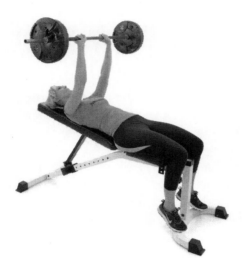

Top Of Movement

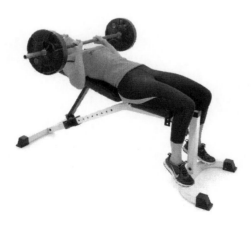

DESCRIPTION OF EXERCISE
CLOSE GRIP BENCH PRESS

Compound exercise targeting: **Rear Upper Arm Muscles**

Start Position: Lay on a bench under a barbell on a rack or smiths machine so that your mid chest is in line with the bar. Take a grip on the bar as you would if you were doing a standard bench press. Now move your grip towards the centre of your body, stopping at shoulder width.

(Some people choose to have an even narrower grip than shoulder width, but as long as you are feeling the exercise on your triceps, your grip width is fine. This seems to be a very personal exercise, so it will pay to experiment with a light weight to find your ideal grip width. In my experience, the longer the trainer's arms, the wider the grip.)

Movement: Lift the bar off the rack or unhook from a smiths machine and straighten your arms, ensuring you do not lock your elbows. As you inhale, lower the bar down to meet your mid chest allowing your elbows to flare out naturally by your sides. As you reach your full range of movement, exhale and push the bar back up to the start position.

You should complete this with a 2-seconds-up-2-seconds-down tempo. This will ensure that you are getting the most out of the exercise.

SHOULDER PRESS

<u>Start Position</u>

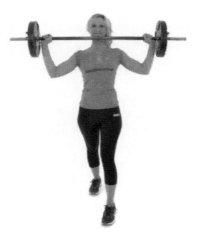

<u>Top Of Movement</u>

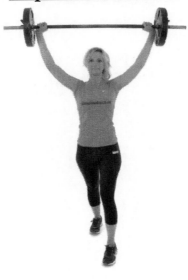

DESCRIPTION OF EXERCISE
SHOULDER PRESS

Compound exercise targeting: **Shoulder Muscles**

Start position: It is best to do these facing a mirror, and, if possible, you should use a rack at shoulder height to hold the barbell before and after sets. Position yourself underneath the barbell on the rack and lift this off, ensuring that your back is straight and the bar does not sink below your chin at any time. Your palms should be facing forwards and hands should be placed about shoulder-width apart.

Movement: As you exhale, push the barbell up above your head to the point just before your elbows lock out. DO NOT ALLOW YOUR ELBOWS TO LOCK OUT AT THE TOP OF THE MOVEMENT. Inhale as you return to the start position.
You should complete this with a 2-seconds-up-2-seconds-down tempo. This will ensure that you are getting the most out of the exercise.

note; please skip this exercise or check with your doctor if you have a known heart condition.

CALF RAISES

Start Position

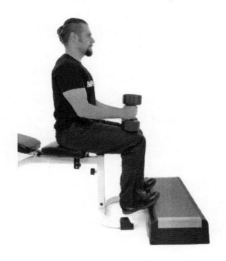

Top Of Movement

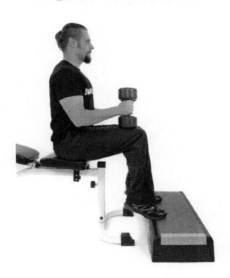

DESCRIPTION OF EXERCISE
CALF RAISES (SEATED)

Exercise targeting: **Lower Rear Leg Muscles (Calves)**

Start position: Sit on a bench and rest the balls of your feet on an exercise step or a raised block. Rest a set of dumbells that allow you to perform your target workload on the lower part of your quads. Keep your toes pointed forward and feet shoulder-width apart whilst ensuring your back is flat.

Movement: As you exhale, raise your heels up as far as you can to feel the squeeze at the top of the movement. (I always hold this position for a second or two, to get the most out of it.) As you inhale, lower your heels back down to where you feel the stretch. It is as important to get a good stretch at the bottom of the movement as the squeeze at the top. Many people neglect this part of the movement.

You should complete this with a 2-seconds-up-2-seconds-down tempo. This will ensure that you are getting the most out of the exercise.

SWISS BALL CRUNCHES

Start Position

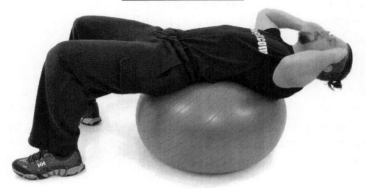

Top Of Movement

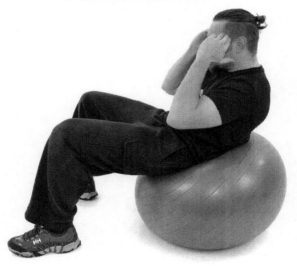

DESCRIPTION OF EXERCISE
SWISS BALL CRUNCHES

Exercise targeting: **Stomach Muscles (Abs)**

Start position: Sit on the swiss ball with your feet flat on the ground. Walk your feet forward so the swiss ball rolls up your back and you are lying in a lying position. The swiss ball should be in your mid to lower back and you should be looking up at the sky. Place your finger tips on the side of your head. DO NOT CLASP YOUR HANDS BEHIND YOUR HEAD.

Movement: Keeping your feet flat on the floor, you should lift your shoulder blades up -- this will put immediate tension on your abdominals. You should breathe out as you do this. Your lower back should not lose contact with the swiss ball and your eyes should be in line with the sky at a 45-degree angle. Once you reach the top of the movement, lower your shoulders to the starting position as you inhale. This completes one rep.

You should complete this with a 2-seconds-up-2-seconds-down tempo. This will ensure that you are getting the most out of the exercise.

DORSAL RAISES

Start Position

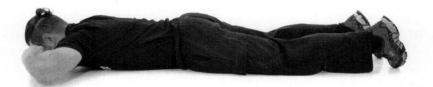

Top Of Movement

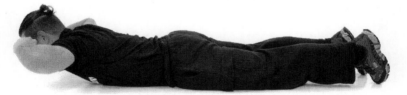

DESCRIPTION OF EXERCISE
DORSAL RAISES

Exercise targeting: **Lower Back Muscles**

Start position: Lay face down on the floor, pointing your toes so the tops of your feet are also in contact with the floor. Your lower arms should be in contact with the floor and at right angles to your upper arms with palms facing down.

Movement: As you breathe out, bring your upper body off the floor, assisting slightly with your hands. Once at the top of the movement, lower your upper body in the same way whilst breathing in. This completes one rep. (It is important to remember that this is a small range of movement so don't strain yourself too much at the top of the movement.)

PUSH UPS

Start Position

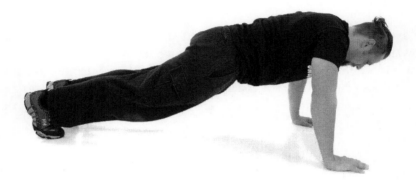

Top Of Movement

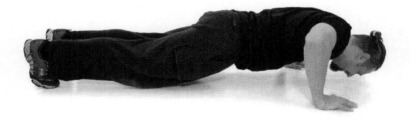

DESCRIPTION OF EXERCISE
PUSH UPS

Exercise targeting: **Chest Muscles**

Start position: Get into a position on the floor so your hands are about shoulder-width apart and in line with your mid/upper chest. You should keep your back flat and take the weight of your body. Make sure that you do not dip your head.

Movement: Keep your back straight and lower your upper body towards the floor by bending your elbows whilst breathing in. Once you are at the bottom of this movement, as you breathe out, raise your upper body back to the starting position. This completes one rep.

SEATED ROWS EXERCISE BAND

Start Position

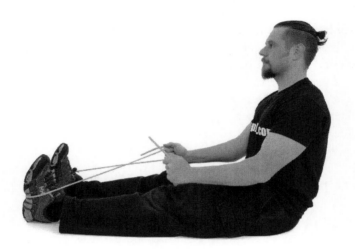

Top Of Movement

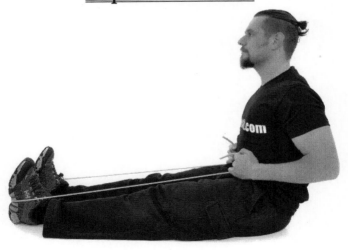

DESCRIPTION OF EXERCISE
SEATED ROWS EXERCISE BAND

Exercise targeting: **Large Back Muscles (Latissimus Dorsi)**

Select an exercise band that will allow you to perform at a challenging but consistent pace throughout the full allocated time of the exercise.

Start position: Sit on the floor with your legs extended out in front of you. Keep your feet together and wrap your exercise band (no attachments) around them. You should ensure that you have equal lengths of exercise band either side of you.

Take hold of the free ends of the exercise band so it is taut. Note that the closer to your feet that you grip the band, the higher the resistance will be. The more that you do this exercise, the easier it will be to know where to grip for your workload.

Whilst in this sitting position and throughout this exercise, you should keep your back straight and keep looking forward.

Movement: Keeping your back straight and torso static, you should pull your fists in to your navel whilst breathing out. During this movement, you should also feel your elbows brush past your lower/mid torso.

At the top of the movement, you can push your chest forward to gain maximum contraction.

Once at the top of the movement, you should breathe in whilst returning to the start position. This completes one rep.

SQUATS

<u>Start Position</u>   <u>Top Of Movement</u>

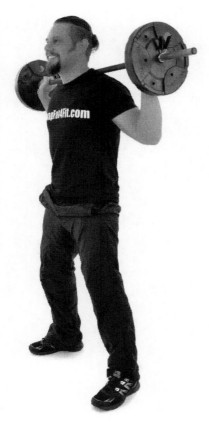
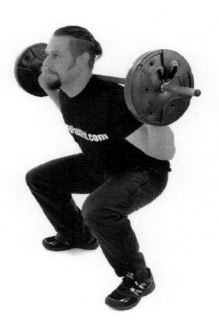

DESCRIPTION OF EXERCISE
SQUATS

Compound exercise targeting: **Upper Leg Muscles**

Start position: Stand with your feet hip-width apart, toes slightly turned out. Take the barbell from the rack by positioning yourself below it and standing up so that the bar rests on your shoulders, ensuring that you keep a flat back. Focus on a point on a wall or in the distance that is eye level or higher and look at this throughout the movement. This will help you keep your posture and maintain correct form.

Movement: Keeping your feet flat on the floor, as you breathe in, bend your knees until your quads (Upper legs) are parallel to the ground. Push back through your heels to the starting position whilst breathing out. Ensure that you are always looking straight ahead or slightly up. This will help you keep a good posture. This completes one rep.

LUNGES

Start Position

Top Of Movement

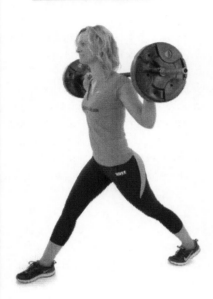
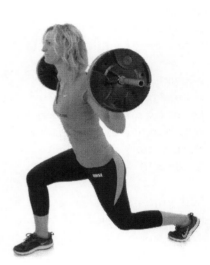

DESCRIPTION OF EXERCISE
LUNGES

Compound exercise targeting: **Upper Leg Muscles**

This is a single leg exercise so when your reach this in your training routine, you should perform this exercise with a set on each leg.

Start position: From a standing position with your feet together, you should take a large step forward with one leg. You should step forward to a point that, when you lunge down, your leading upper leg forms a right angle with your leading lower leg.

Once you have established this distance, you should stand up, keeping your feet planted in this position. Your toes on both feet should be pointing forward and your legs should not move laterally from your hip joint. Because you will have a narrow stance, you should counter balance with your arms if needed. This may be hard at first, but even balancing in this position is developing stabilizer muscles in your body.

Movement: From this standing position, keep your back flat, feet planted in the stated position and head looking directly forward. As you inhale, lower yourself down by lunging until your knee is just about to touch the floor, but do not let your knee rest on the ground. Once at the top of this movement, return to the start position as you exhale, ensuring your feet do not shift.

CLOSE GRIP PUSHUPS

Start Position

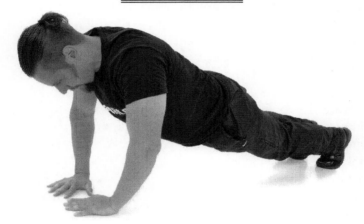

Top Of Movement

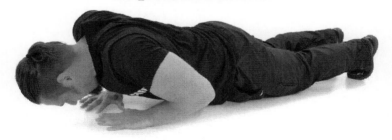

DESCRIPTION OF EXERCISE
CLOSE GRIP PUSHUPS

Exercise targeting: **Upper rear arm muscles (triceps)**

Start position: Take a position on the floor so that you are on your hands and knees. Draw your hands in towards the center of your body in line with your mid chest. Your hands should be at least shoulder-width apart. People with shorter arms may want to bring their hands even closer together. From this position, push your legs back and take the weight of your body on your toes and hands. Ensure that your back is flat at this point and throughout the movement.

Movement: Keeping your back flat, lower your body by bending your arms to a point where your nose is about to touch the floor. You should breath in as you lower yourself. As you exhale, return to the starting position.
You should complete this with a 2-seconds-up-2-seconds-down tempo. This will ensure that you are getting the most out of the exercise.

LATERAL RAISES WITH DUMBBELLS

Start Position

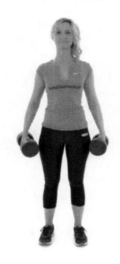

Top Of Movement

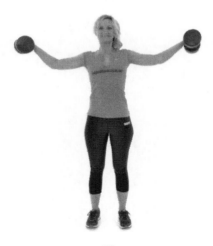

DESCRIPTION OF EXERCISE
LATERAL RAISES WITH DUMBBELLS

Exercise targeting: **Shoulder Muscles (Delts)**

Start position: It's best to do this sitting on a bench, although it can be performed standing up. You should use an adjustable bench and set this so it is just under maximum upright position (1 notch back). Grab your dumbbells and sit on the bench. Allow your arms to hang down by your sides with your palms facing inwards. Keep your elbows slightly bent.

Movement: As you exhale, raise your arms so they are parallel to the ground and out to your sides. The only joint that should be moving here is your shoulder. Inhale as you lower to the start position.
You should complete this with a 2-seconds-up-2-seconds-down tempo. This will ensure that you are getting the most out of the exercise.

PUSH UPS ON KNEES

Start Position

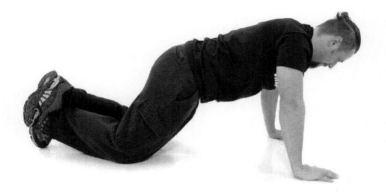

Top Of Movement

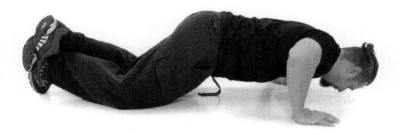

DESCRIPTION OF EXERCISE
PUSH UPS ON KNEES

Start position: Get to a position on the floor so you are on your hands and knees.

Your hands should be about shoulder-width apart and in line with your face.

Movement: Keep your back straight and lower your upper body towards the floor by bending your elbows and breathing in.

Once you are at the bottom of this movement, whilst breathing out, raise your upper body back to the starting position. This completes one rep. If you can do more than 30, move to full push ups.

STEP UPS

Stage 1

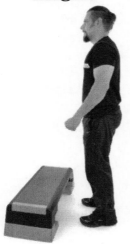

Stage 2

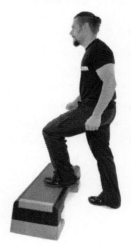

Stage 3

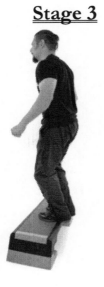

Stage 4

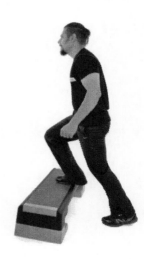

DESCRIPTION OF EXERCISE
STEP UPS

Start position: Set up an exercise step or something similar. And stand on the floor in front of the equipment.

Mid position: This is a step up, step down movement and used for the "active rest" sets on a circuit training routine. Simply step up with one foot at a time until you have both feet on the step. At this point, you should step down leading with the foot you used first to step onto the step. When performing this exercise, you should set the pace so that it is still challenging but you can perform the exercise comfortably for your allocated time slot.

You should also concentrate on your breathing. Try to find a regular pattern as soon as you start the exercise.

BODYWEIGHT SQUATS

Start Position

Top Of Movement

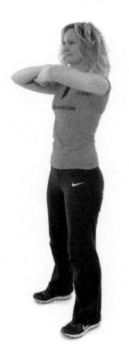

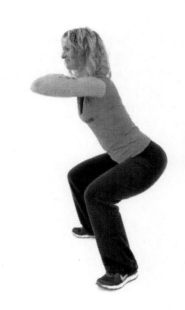

DESCRIPTION OF EXERCISE
BODYWEIGHT SQUATS

Exercise targeting: **Upper Legs**

Start position: Stand with your feet hip-width apart, toes slightly turned out and your arms across your chest. Focus on a point on a wall or in the distance that is eye level or higher and look at this throughout the movement. This will help you keep your posture and maintain correct form.

Movement: Keeping your feet flat on the floor, as you breathe in, bend your knees until your quads (Upper legs) are parallel to the ground. Push back through your heels to the starting position, whilst breathing out. Ensure that you are always looking straight ahead or slightly up. This will help you keep a good posture. This completes one rep.

TRICEP DIPS

Start Position

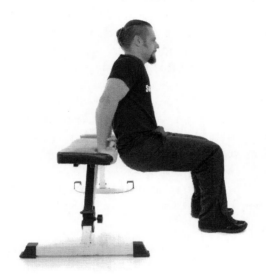

Top Of Movement

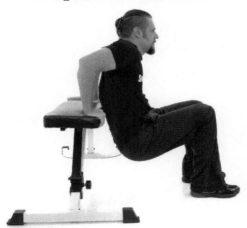

DESCRIPTION OF EXERCISE
TRICEP DIPS

Exercise targeting: **Rear Upper Arms (Triceps)**

Start position: Sit on a bench or chair, put your hands palm down and flat on the bench by your sides so they are in line with your shoulders (If this is uncomfortable, try moving your hands to a wider position). Take the weight of your body onto your arms. Ensure that your arms are not locked out; you should have them slightly bent. Your feet should be flat on the floor out in front of you.

Movement: As you inhale, lower your body down by bending your elbows. You should lower yourself so that your upper arms are parallel to the ground. As you exhale, return to the starting position by straightening your arms. Remember; DO NOT LOCK YOUR ARMS AT THE TOP OF THIS MOVEMENT.
You should complete this with a 2-seconds-up-2-seconds-down tempo. This will ensure that you are getting the most out of the exercise.

SHOULDER PRESS
(EXERCISE BANDS)

Start Position

Top Of Movement

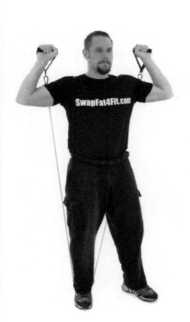

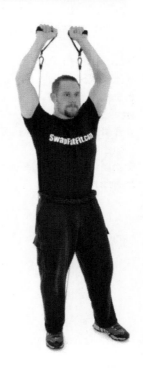

DESCRIPTION OF EXERCISE
SHOULDER PRESS (EXERCISE BANDS)

Exercise targeting: **Shoulders (Deltoids)**

Attach stirrups to each end of the band.

Start position: Hold a stirrup in each hand, step forward with one foot securing the middle of the band under the rear foot. Keep your palms facing forward and in line with your chin. Your eyes should be looking straight and your back should be flat.

Movement: Whilst breathing out and maintaining your posture, push the stirrups above your head as high as you can, bringing the two stirrups together to touch at the top of the movement. You should not let your elbows lock. As you breathe in, lower your arms back to the starting position. This completes one rep.

*note; please skip this exercise or check with your doctor if you have a known heart condition.

CRUNCHES

Start Position

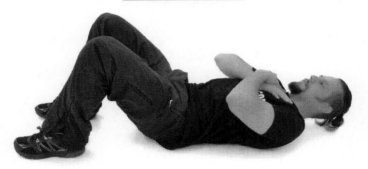

Top Of Movement

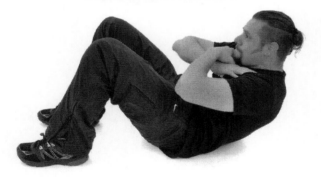

DESCRIPTION OF EXERCISE
CRUNCHES

Start position: Lay flat on your back and bring your knees up so that your feet are flat on the floor about shoulder-width apart. Place the tips of your fingers on the side of your head or cross your hands across your chest.
DO NOT CLASP YOUR HANDS BEHIND YOUR HEAD.

Movement: As you breathe out, slowly lift your upper body off the floor, bending at your hips. Once at the top of this movement, breathe in as you lower your upper body back to the start position. This completes one rep.

BENCH JUMPS

Start Position

Top Of Movement

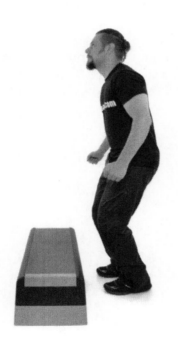
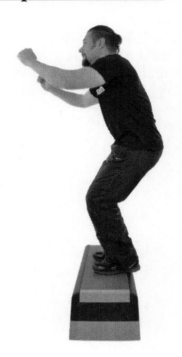

DESCRIPTION OF EXERCISE
BENCH JUMPS

Start position: Set up an exercise step or something similar (the higher the step or platform you decide to use, the more challenging the exercise will become). Stand on the floor in front of the equipment.

Mid position: From a stationary position with both feet together, simply take a two-footed jump onto the step. Both of your feet should make contact with the step at the same time. Once on the step, immediately step down and assume the starting position again. Try to keep the movement continuous throughout your allocated set time. It will help if you find a rhythm with the cadence of the exercise and your breathing.

ALTERNATE SQUAT THRUSTS

Stage 1

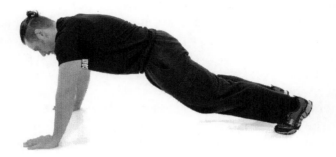

Stage 2

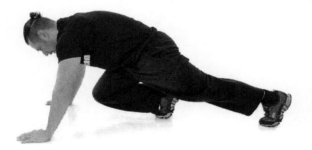

Stage 3

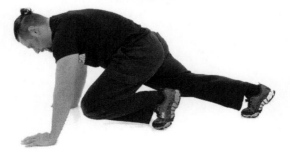

DESCRIPTION OF EXERCISE
ALTERNATE SQUAT THRUSTS

Note: This is a "dynamic" or "Plyometric" exercise, which means that it will be done at a fairly fast pace and can be quiet intense. So please keep this in mind on performance.

Start position: Get into a position on the floor so your hands are about shoulder-width apart and in line with your mid/upper chest. You should keep your back flat and take the weight of your body. Make sure that you do not dip your head. This is the same starting position as pushups.

Movement: Whilst keeping a regular breathing pattern, you should "shoot" one of your legs up towards your chest while the other stays extended. Almost immediately after the toes of the moving leg hit the floor, in one motion, you should "shoot" it back to the starting position whilst simultaneously "shooting" the other leg towards your chest.

This exercise should flow and you should be constantly moving throughout your exercise time slot.

CRAWLING STEPS

<u>Stage 1</u>

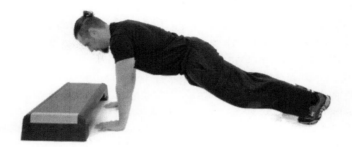

<u>Stage 2</u>

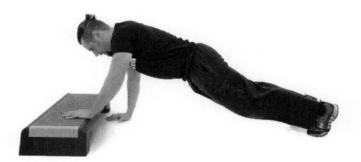

<u>Stage 3</u>

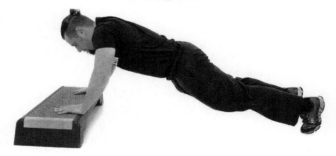

DESCRIPTION OF EXERCISE
CRAWLING STEPS

Start position: Place an exercise step on the ground. You may want to butt this up against a wall or other solid object as it may shift whilst you are performing the exercise.

In front of this step, get into a position on the floor so your hands are about shoulder-width apart and in line with your mid/upper chest. You should keep your back flat and take the weight of your body. Make sure that you do not dip your head. This is the same starting position as pushups.

Movement: From the start position, place one hand onto the step and as soon as you have taken your body weight with this hand, immediately follow with your other hand. As soon as you have both hands on the step, place your first hand back onto the floor. Immediately follow with your second hand. As soon as you have both hands on the floor, you should start the process again.

It is important to maintain a steady consistent breathing pattern when performing this exercise.

This exercise should flow and you should be constantly moving throughout your exercise time slot.

STAR JUMPS

Start Position

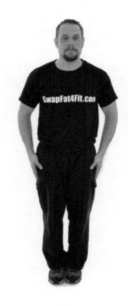

Top Of Movement

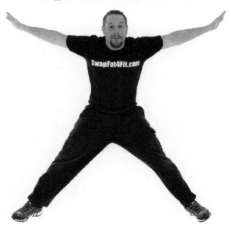

DESCRIPTION OF EXERCISE
STAR JUMPS

Note: This is a "dynamic" or "Plyometric" exercise, which means that it will be done at a fairly fast pace and can be quiet intense. So please keep this in mind on performance.

Start position: Stand up straight with your feet and knees together. Your hands and arms should be in contact with your body

Movement: As you exhale, jump into the air, raising your arms so they reach at least parallel to the floor whilst simultaneously moving your feet in the same direction.
On landing, your feet and knees should be in the start position along with your hands and arms.

CHAPTER 17

OUTRO

I hope that this book has been useful. As you can see, there can be a pretty diverse approach to superset training and indeed resistance training in general.

If you have a better understanding of how to incorporate this training method into your own personal fitness journey after reading this book, then I am a "happy ted", as this is what I set out to do.

One thing that I would like to point out again is that the theories and exercise routines that are outlined in this book are my own creation, based on my education in the health and fitness field and also on my personal experiences.

I wish you every success with your training and I hope that you hit all of your fitness goals.

All the best,

Jim.

CHAPTER 18

I WILL LEAVE YOU WITH THIS

There are many ways in which you can progress in the fitness world. There are lots of different routes that you can travel down. For instance, someone starting out may decide that they want to become more muscle bound and favor the resistance training side of fitness over the cardiovascular side.

Everyone will have a different story. The next chapter is an excerpt from one of my other books. It is my story of becoming a long distance runner. If you do feel that you would like to take up running and work on your cardio vascular and fat burning fitness potential, why not learn from my mistakes and personal experience?

You will always get to where you want to be a whole lot quicker if you learn from someone else's mistakes.

CHAPTER 19

MARATHON TRAINING AND DISTANCE RUNNING TIPS

I know there are plenty of books out there about this type of training, but I would like to share my firsthand experience of developing from a guy who couldn't run 1.5 miles in 15 minutes to a guy who could be handed a pair of running shoes and be standing confidently at the start line of a marathon in the time it took to tie those shoes up. That was all the preparation time that I needed.

Oh, and I got to a point when I could cover the same 1.5 mile distance in 8 minutes and 22 seconds!

Let's start at the beginning.

It was the summer of 1999, and I had just finished my secondary school education. Not being an academic and not knowing what I wanted to do with my life, I decided to enrol for a Business Studies class at college. It wasn't long before I realised that sitting in an office was not something that I really wanted to do. (Looking back, this was a fairly good opportunity, but *you live, you learn*, I suppose.)

Anyway, about six months into this college education, I decided that I wanted a bit of excitement from my life and the thought of being an average Joe with a regular nine-to-five job made me pretty depressed. It was at this point that I ventured into the local army careers office.

"So, do you have any idea what you want to do as a job in the army?" asked the sergeant at the front desk.

I had heard a lot about airborne forces and the parachute regiment and wanted a piece of that.

"Yeah. I want to look at joining the paras," I said, not realising at that time that you don't simply "join the paras!"

"Okay, let's have a chat," he replied (probably thinking, "Jeez! Here's another one with absolutely no clue!")

The sergeant had a good chat with me and concluded that I should look at getting a trade in the Royal Engineers; I could then volunteer for para training at a later date. This way I would have a trade, be on higher pay, and also get to jump out of planes and serve with airborne forces.

To go down this path, however, I would need to pass the aptitude test at a higher level.

I took this aptitude test four times with a six-week gap between tests before the sergeant just gave me a pass. (I actually think I failed the fourth time as well, but he just fixed my score. It was good to see someone give me a chance.)

So that was me going to the next stage of the army selection process. And this was the fitness testing stage!

These fitness tests were over a long weekend where all potential recruits are taken to an army training centre and tested on attitude, strength, and endurance and checked if we were medically fit.

As I was into weight training at the time, I did well with the strength tests, but, on the last day, there is a mile-and-a-half run that must be completed in something like fifteen minutes. This is very achievable and you could probably do this at a fast-paced walk.

This circuit is led by a PTI (physical training instructor) who is the pace maker. If you stick with this guy, you will pass—simple!

There were about twenty guys on this stage of the selection process with me, and we all started at a steady jog close to the PTI. At about a minute into the test, my breathing was all over the place, my lower back was giving me pain, and I started to get a stitch. I must have looked like I was at the final few miles of a marathon! I remember the PTI turning to me and shouting,

"What's up, Atkinson? You got a sucking chest wound?" before laughing and leaving me to drop back behind the whole squad.

When I eventually crossed the finish line, I gave my name to one of the corporals and he noted my time down. Needless to say, this was a big fat fail, and if I did want to join the army, I would have to start some kind of running programme.

Back at the careers office, the same sergeant that I had originally spoken to gave me a fitness plan to follow so I could try again in six months' time.

So getting into the army wasn't as easy as I had first thought, and I was glad that I had been put on the "trade path" rather than the "parachute regiment path" at this point.

College was still in the picture, and I would get up an hour earlier each morning and run around a two-mile circuit that I had planned out. At first, this took 25 minutes, and within a few weeks, it was down to seventeen minutes—sorted!

The time came for the next selection process, and I flew through it, sticking with the PTI and being amongst the first to cross the finish line on the final mile and a half test.

I finally joined the army in 2001, so this had taken me the best part of two years!

ONE LAST THING

I would like to take this opportunity to send you a sincere "thank you" for purchasing this book. It really means a lot to me that you chose this over all of the other competition.

I would also like to let you know that this book is self-published. This means that I have had no help with promotion or financial backing in the writing, editing, design and publishing processes of this book.

I strongly believe that this is a very good guide and I would like to get it into the hands of as many people in need of real weight loss and fitness help as possible.

Therefore, I would be delighted if you would mention this to your friends if you think that they will benefit from it. Facebook it, tweet it, blog it! ☺

Many thanks, good luck and I look forward to hearing from you!

All the very best,

Jim.

ALSO BY JAMES ATKINSON

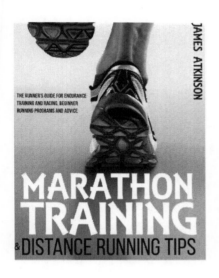

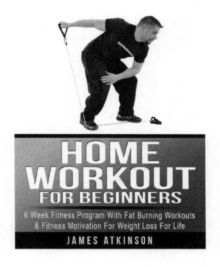

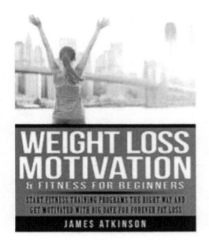

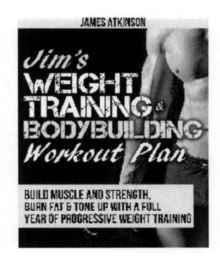

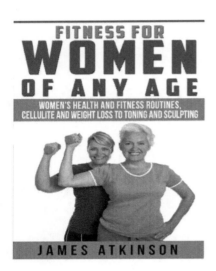

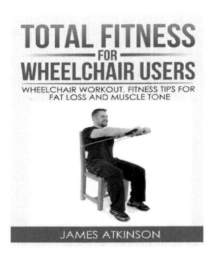

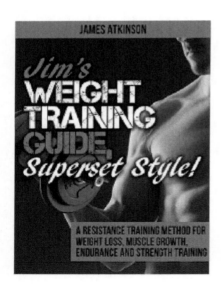

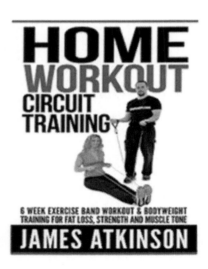

CONNECT WITH JIM

Visit Jim's blog for more great advice on diet, training, healthy recipes, motivation and more: www.jimshealthandmuscle.com

Get regular updates on Facebook when you "like" and "follow" Jim's pages here:

Facebook.com/JimsHealthandMuscle
Facebook.com/SwapFat4Fit

Catch the trends. Follow Jim on Twitter here:

@JimsHM

Printed in Great Britain
by Amazon.co.uk, Ltd.,
Marston Gate.